Better Than a Pink Ribbon:
A kid's guide to their parent's cancer

Gabriel Insler

2015

First Printing: 2015

ISBN 978-0-692-76570-8

Gabriel Insler
9 Orchard Ave.
Providence, RI 02906

This Book is Dedicated to MY Mom,

The person who inspired me to write this Book.

HI! My name is Gabe Insler and I am currently 13 years old. My mom was diagnosed with cancer in February 2013, and it was hard. As a project, I decided to do something good for kids who are going through the same thing that I went through and help them understand what is happening to them, and their parents. This book includes the reasoning behind the mind of a parent, and mom pages, which are actual quotes from my mom, saying how she feels and what is going on in her head. Because this book is written by me, ... a kid, I will not be using too many scientific terms and things like that. But I will be sharing my own personal opinions and experiences on the matter. Now, please, OPEN UP THE BOOK AND SEE WHAT'S INSIDE!

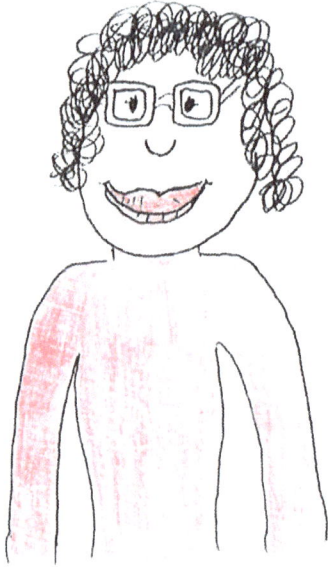

MOM, WOMAN OF MYSTERY...

THOUGHTS FINALLY REVEALED!

SO YOUR PARENT HAS CANCER?

SO DID MINE!

IF YOU ARE AS SCARED AND WORRIED AS
I WAS, THIS BOOK IS FOR
YOU!

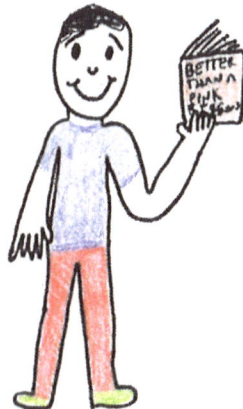

BUT DON'T WORRY!
I'M HERE TO HELP!

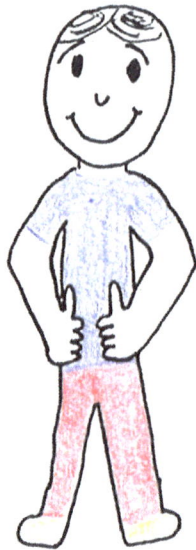

WHEN YOU HEAR THAT YOUR PARENT HAS
CANCER, ONE OF
THE FIRST QUESTIONS YOU MIGHT ASK IS,...

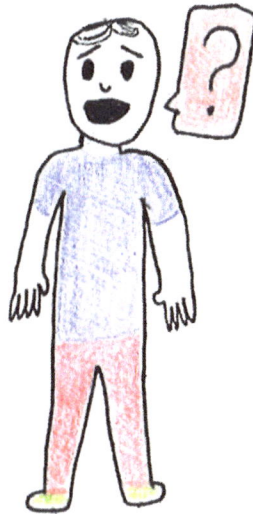

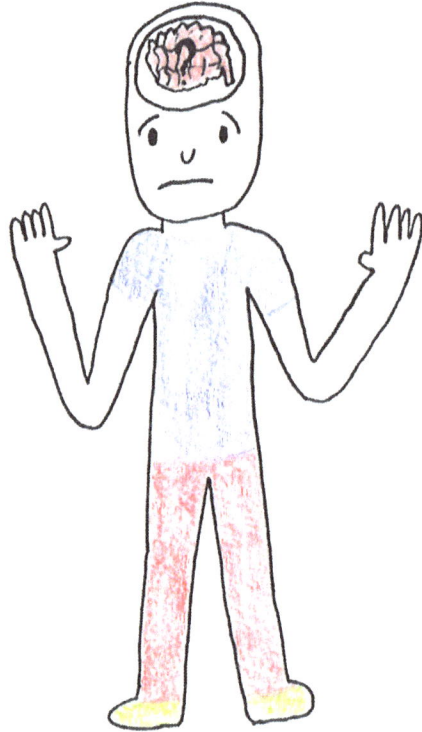

IMAGINE THAT THE CELL HAS THE FLU, AND IT IS GETTING EVERYONE ELSE AROUND IT SICK.

FROM THIS...

TO THIS...

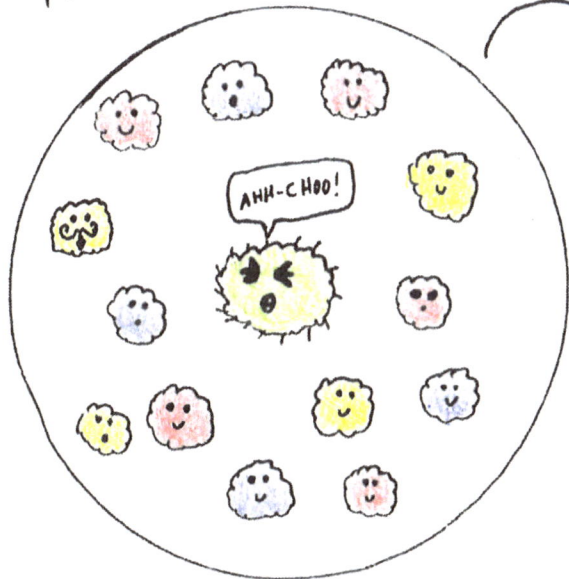

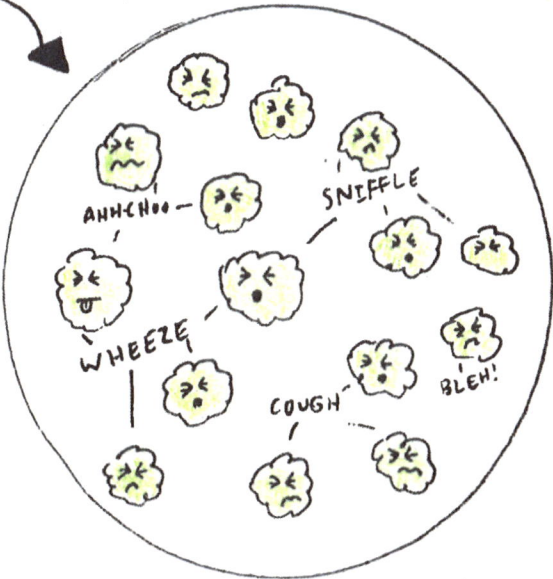

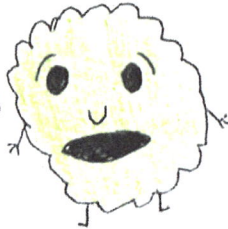

WHEN YOUR PARENT TELLS YOU THAT THEY
HAVE CANCER, DO NOT

FLIP OUT !!!!!

CANCER CREATES A DIFFICULT AND STRESSFUL
ENVIRONMENT
IN THE HOUSE.

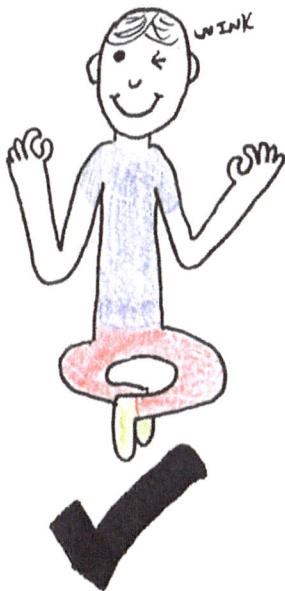

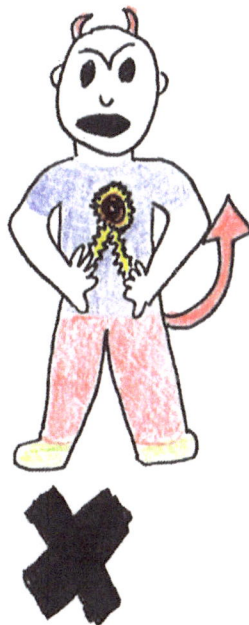

YOUR PARENT IS JUST AS SCARED AND WORRIED ABOUT WHAT IS TO COME AS YOU ARE.

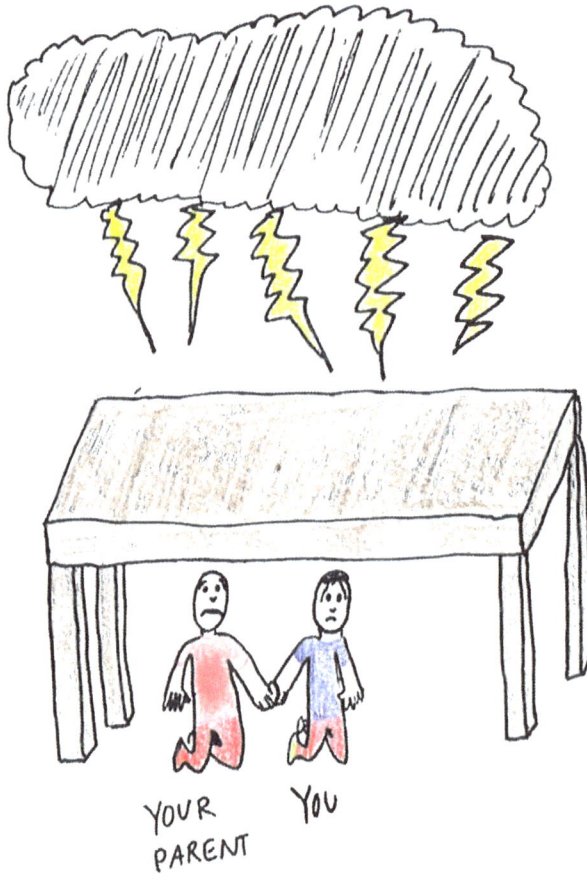

YOUR PARENT   YOU

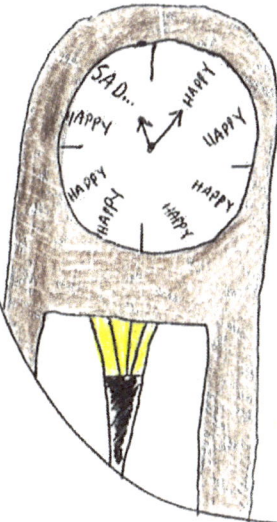

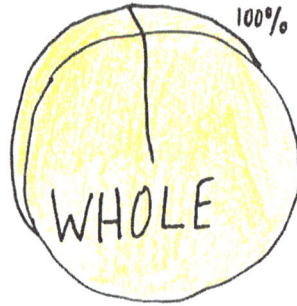

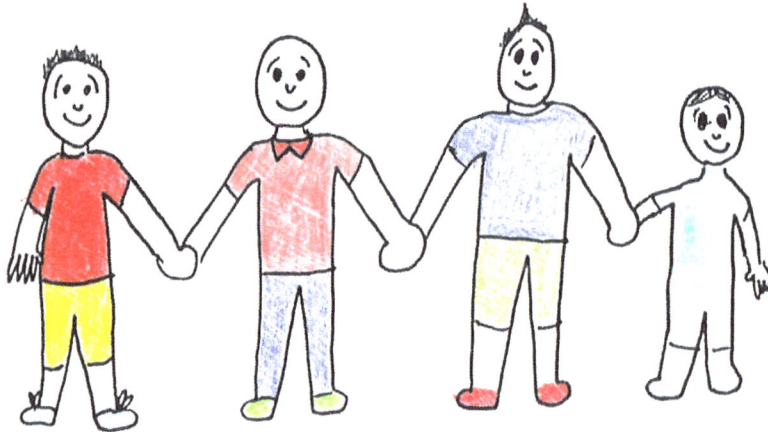

ONCE YOUR PARENT IS DIAGNOSED WITH
CANCER, A LOT

OF THINGS ARE GOING TO CHANGE.

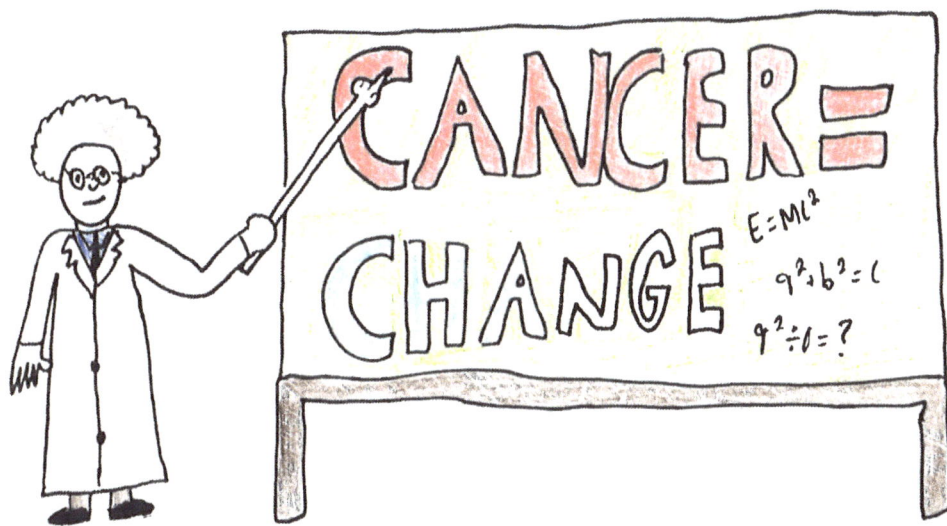

YOU MIGHT GET MORE PLAYDATES, MORE RESPONSIBILITY, MORE

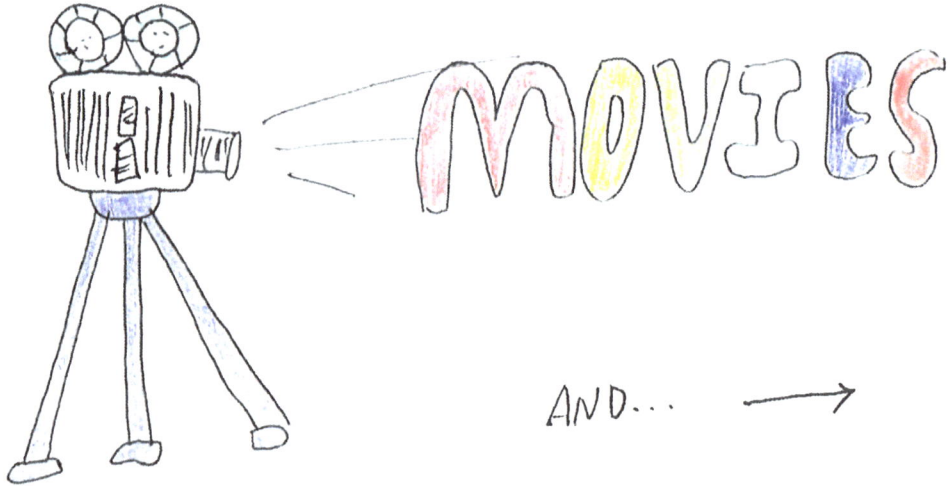

MOVIES

AND... →

MORE ICE CREAM!! :)

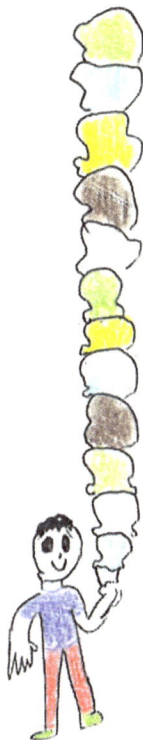

I am working hard at being healthy,
but that's not my whole world.

You are.

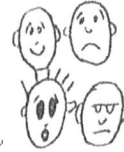

I want to know everything:
if you are happy, scared, grumpy, excited,
about the book you are reading
school, sports practice, your friends ...
it's okay to talk
(and think) about
not cancer stuff.

mom

MY MOM WANTED THESE WEIRD

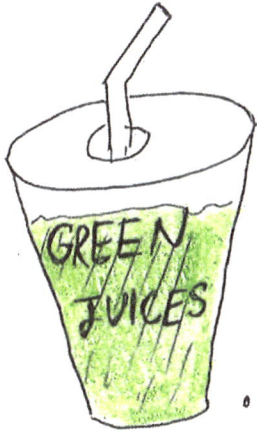

THEY ARE MADE WITH LIKE

1,000,000,000,000,000,000 Vegetables!

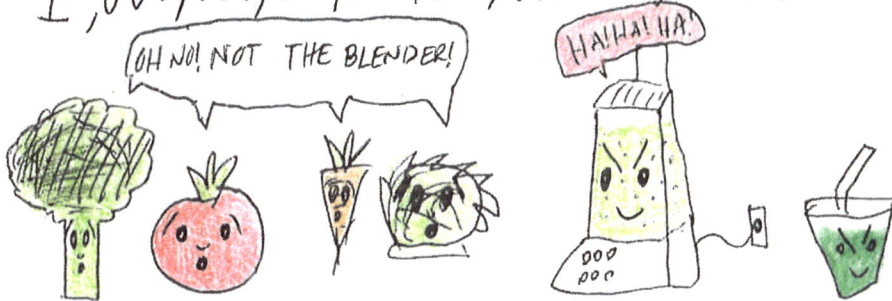

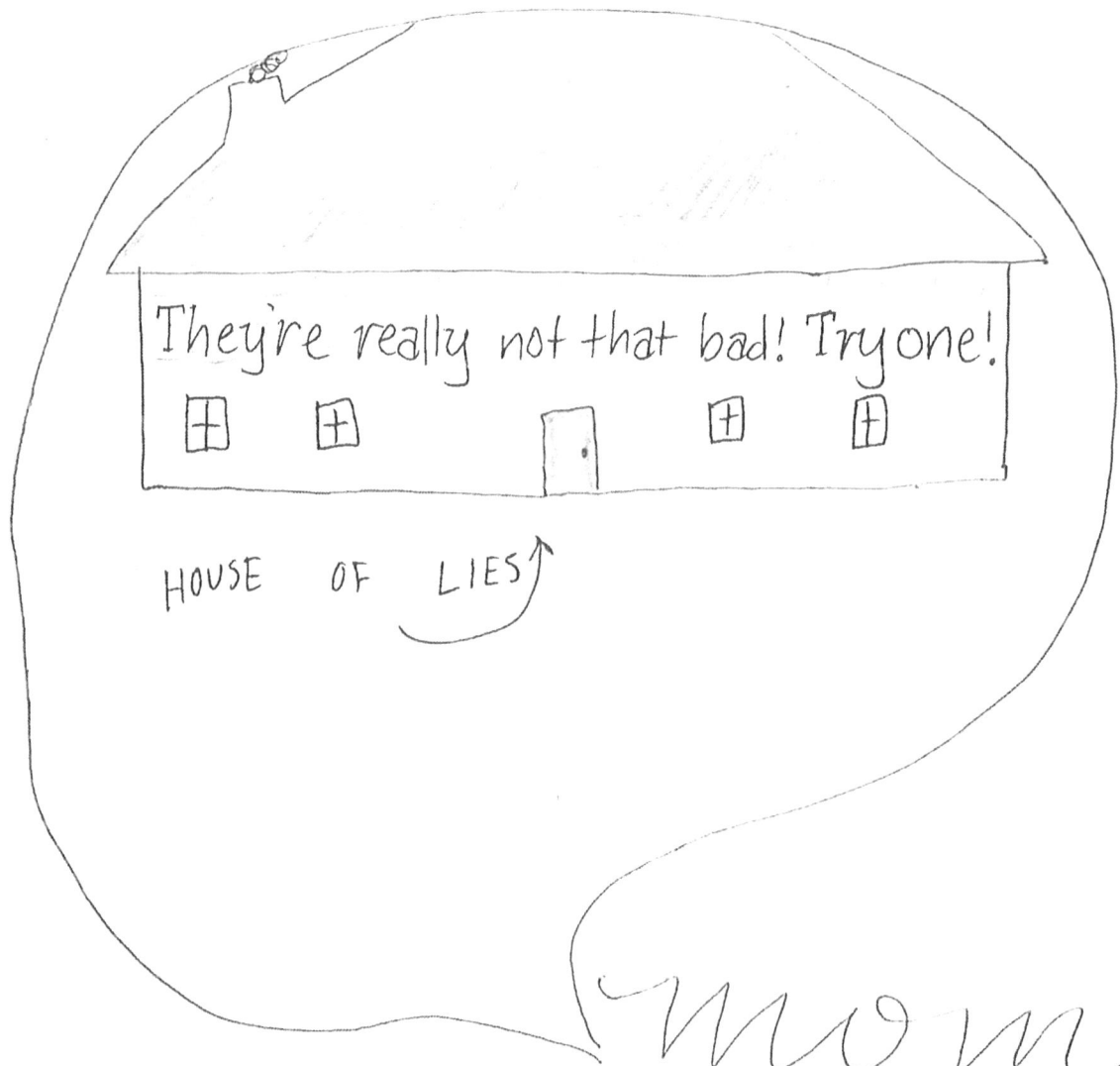

BE WARNED! NO MATTER WHAT ANYONE SAYS, THEY ARE DISGUSTING!

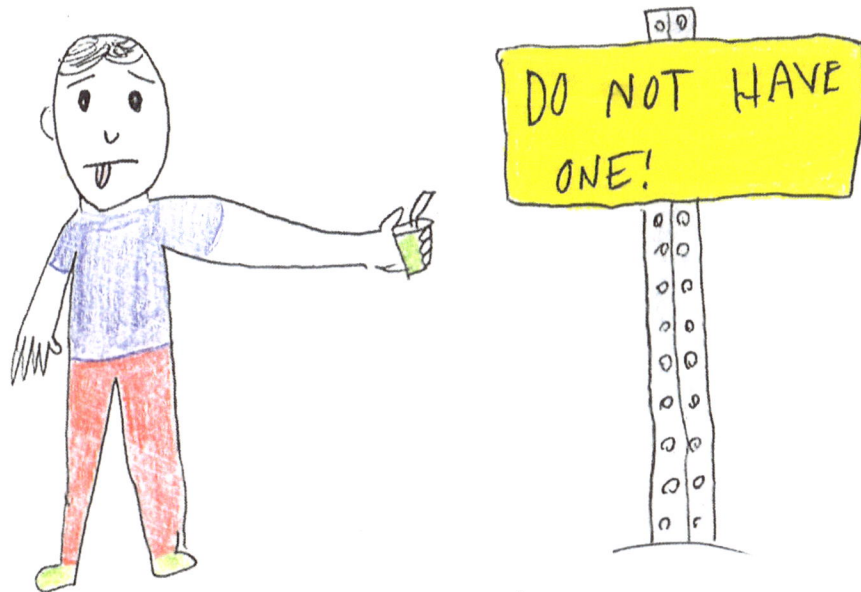

BUT THE ONLY REASON THAT THEY ARE
GIVING YOU THIS STUFF
IS FOR YOUR

H E A L T H

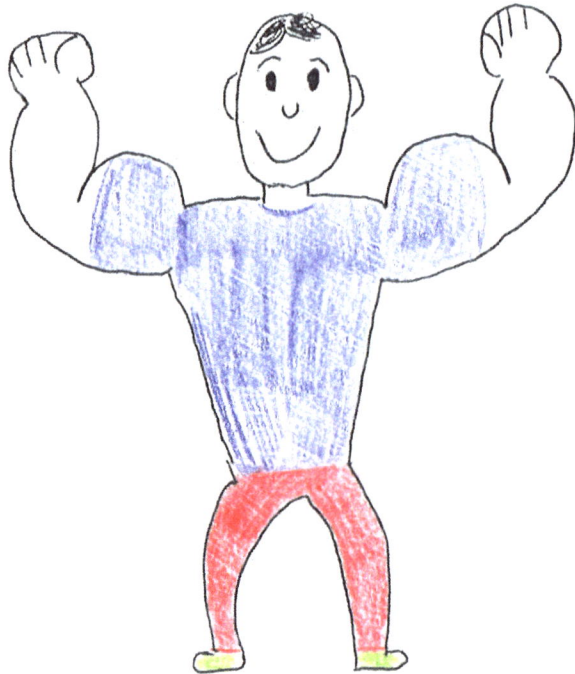

YOUR PARENT MIGHT TAKE AWAY SOME THINGS LIKE

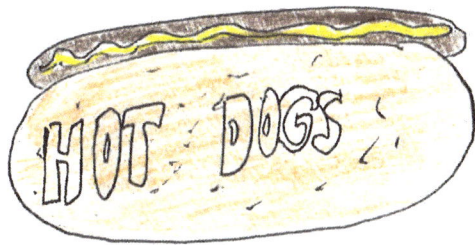 OR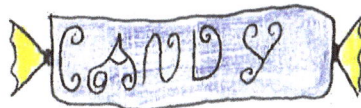

YOUR PARENT

STEALTH MODE

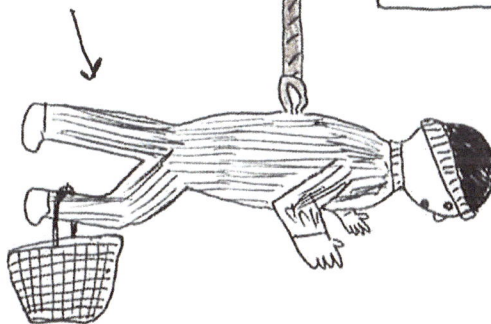

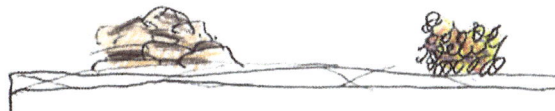

YOUR PARENT IS NOT DOING THESE THINGS TO BE

MEAN and TERRIBLE.

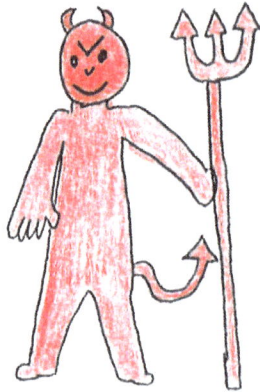
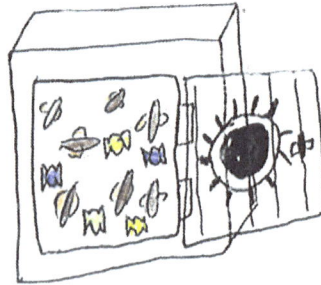

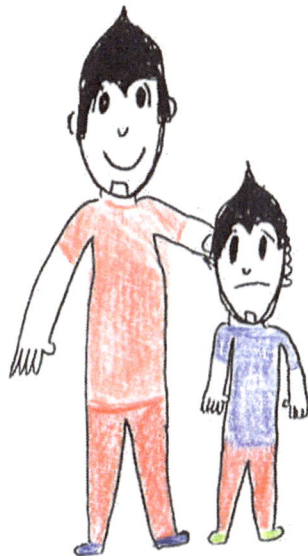

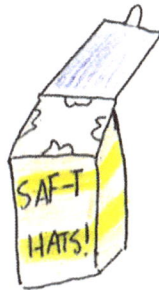

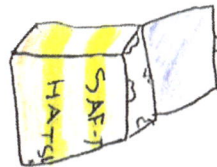

Because cancer runs in my family,

I believe we should take good care of
ourselves and
STACK THE DECK in our favor.

Fuel our bodies with health!

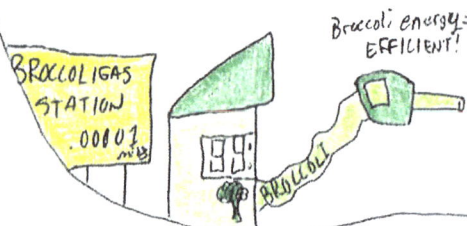

Broccoli energy=
EFFICIENT!

BROCCOLI GAS
STATION
.00001
mi$

BROCCOLI

mom

YOU SHOULD SPEND TIME WITH YOUR PARENT! (T.V., Games, Reading, etc.)

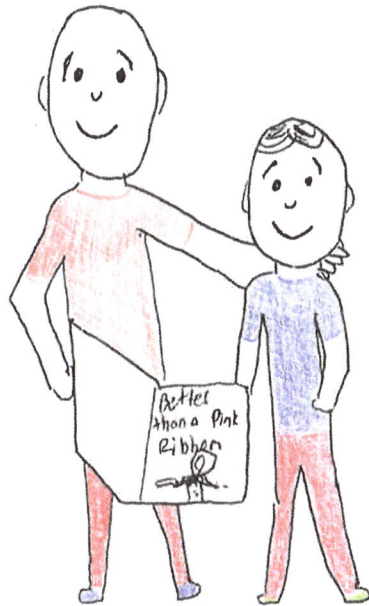

THIS WILL HELP YOUR PARENT

RECUPERATE = FASTER

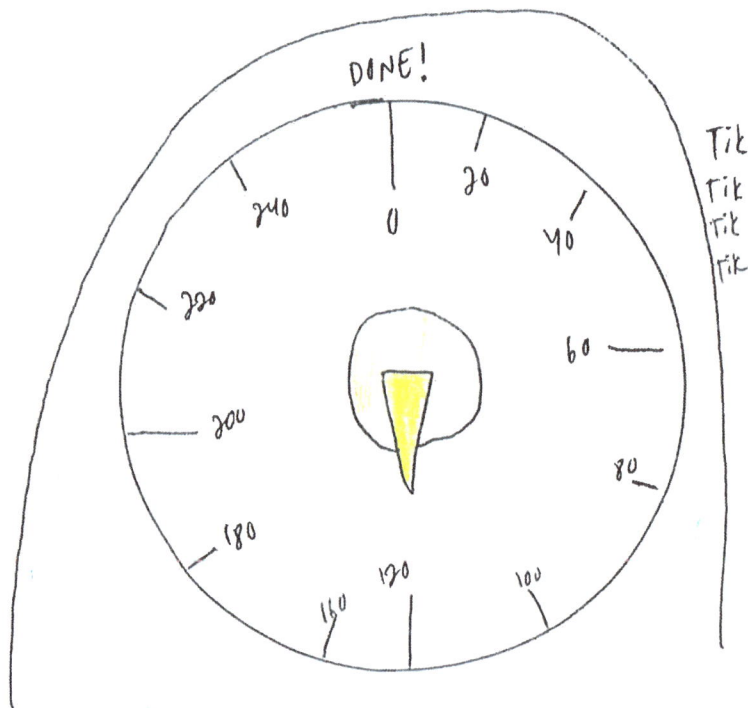

DONE!

240   0   20   40

220   60

200   80

180   100

160   120   100

Tik
Tik
Tik
Tik

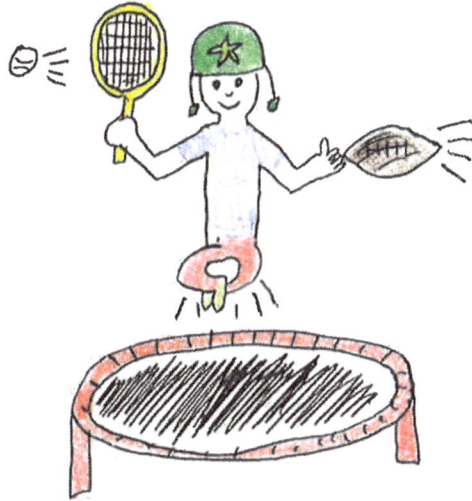

TELLING PEOPLE CAN BE HARD,
BUT PEOPLE ARE NICER THAN YOU THINK
THEY WILL BE.

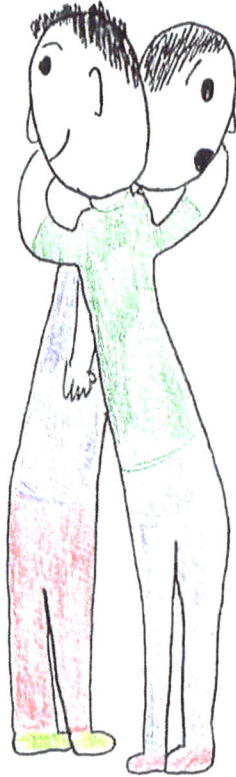

OVER SYMPATHY FEELS WEIRD KNOWING THAT MY MOM IS SUPER STRONG and could handle it. HAVING PEOPLE PITY HER FELT STRANGE.

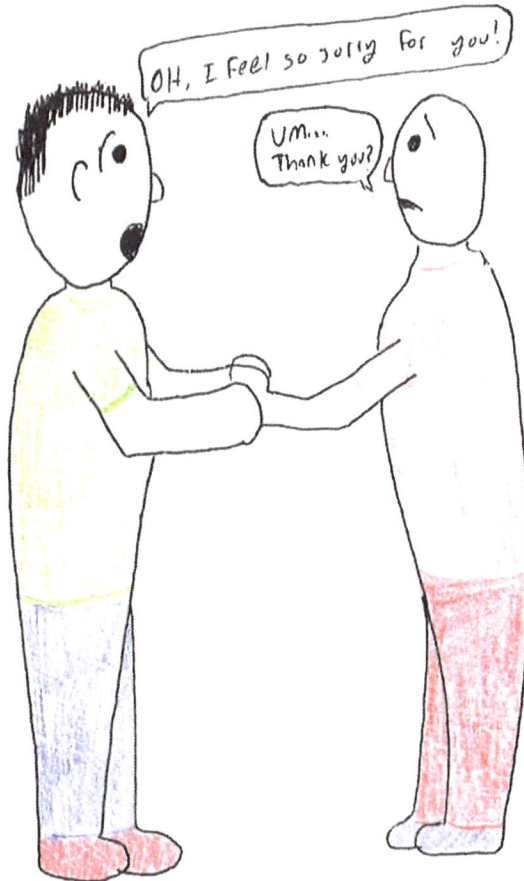

During Breast Cancer Awareness Month, a lot of people at my school wore pink clothes and pink ribbons because they were being "aware". Just being "aware" doesn't do anything.

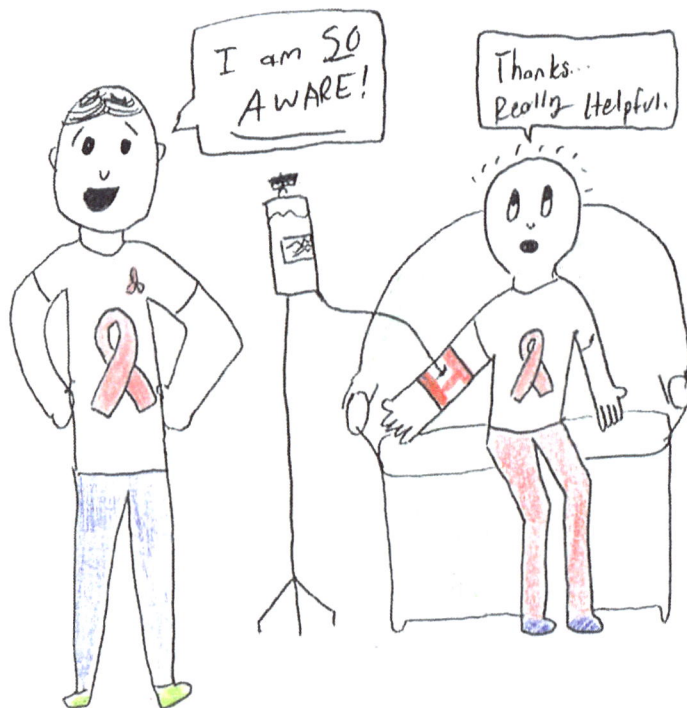

Also during Cancer Awareness Month, you might feel like you are different or someone standing out in a croud, but it helps to group together with your friends. If you want to make a big difference, you can ask some of your friends to donate 💵 to a cancer cause.

Money

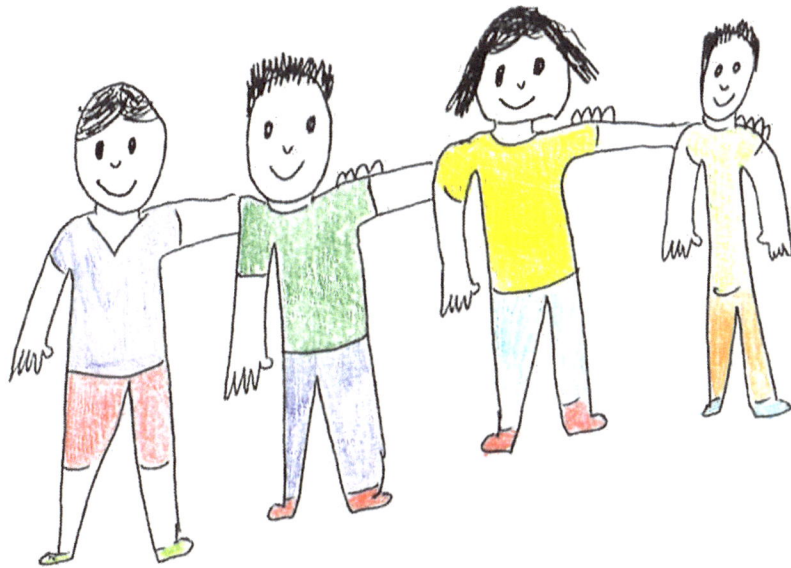

If you are curious and don't know how to act or behave around your diagnosed parent, you shouldn't be worried.

NO MORE OF THIS!

Ah, Um, well, you see... um.

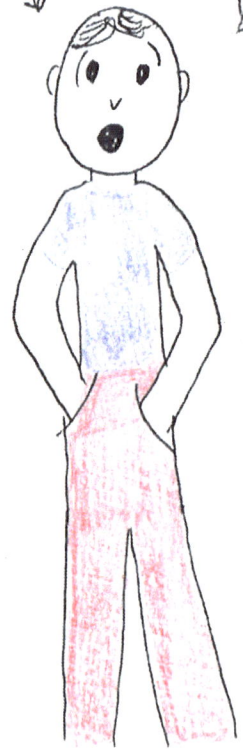

It is not much different from how you would treat your parent any other day, just with a little more -

° HELPFULNESS

° KINDNESS

AND

° CONSIDERATION

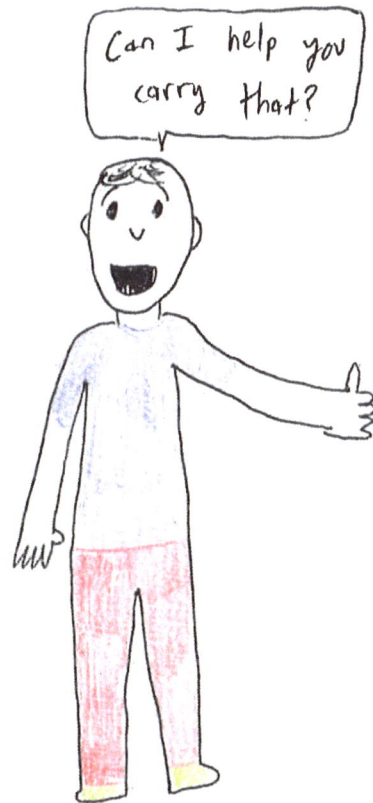

Can I help you carry that?

IF YOUR PARENT FEELS SLEEPY,
LET THEM REST! THEY NEED TO
REGAIN THEIR STRENGTH!

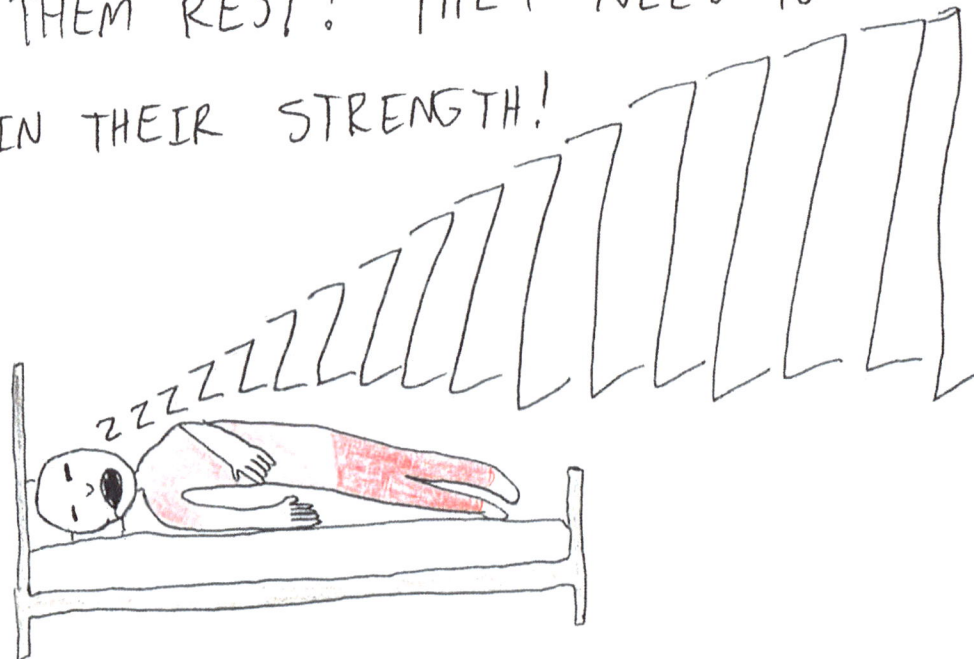

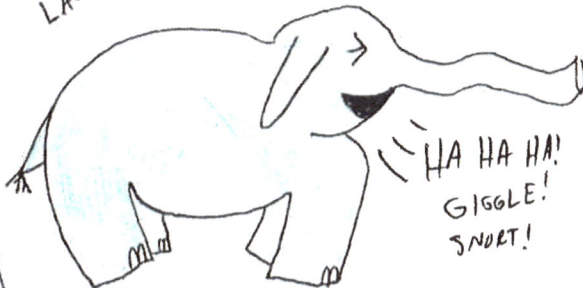

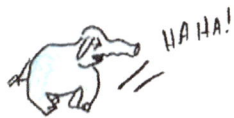

DON'T BE AFRAID TO TALK TO YOUR PARENT ABOUT YOUR WORRIES AND FEARS. THEY WILL BE GLAD TO DISCUSS IT WITH YOU.

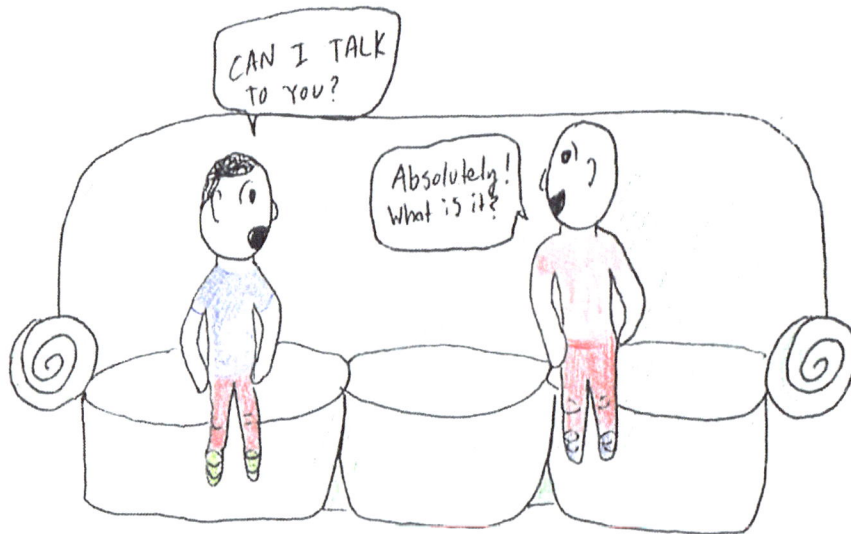

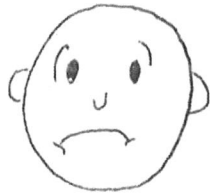

THERE ARE A LOT OF DIFFERENT TREATMENTS FOR CANCER, SOME OF THEM ARE-

- CHEMOTHERAPY

- RADIATION

- PILLS & MEDICINE

- SURGERY

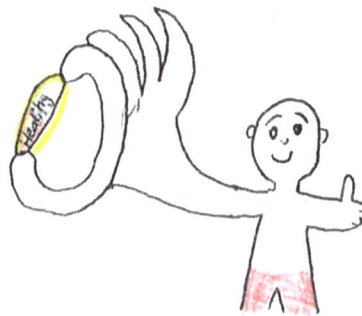

YOUR PARENT MIGHT HAVE SOME SIDE
EFFECTS FROM THE MEDICINE LIKE

- BALDNESS,

- CHANGE OF SKIN COLOR OR

- WEIRD GROSS NAILS

  THESE THINGS MAY HAPPEN,
  BUT YOUR PARENT IS STILL
  YOUR PARENT!

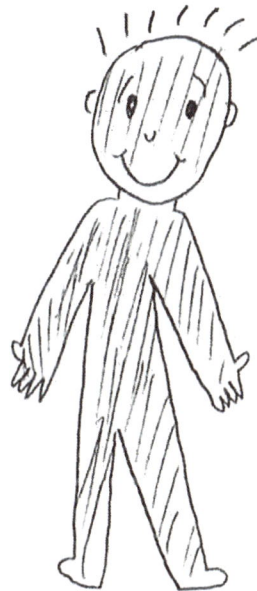

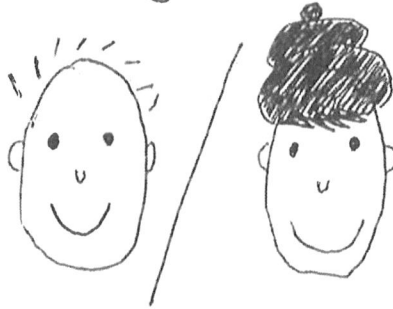

YOU MAY START TO NOTICE WOMEN WEARING SCARVES and 🎩 🎓 🧢 🧕 THAT YOU NEVER NOTICED BEFORE. THERE ARE MANY, MANY OTHER PEOPLE GOING THROUGH CANCER TOO.

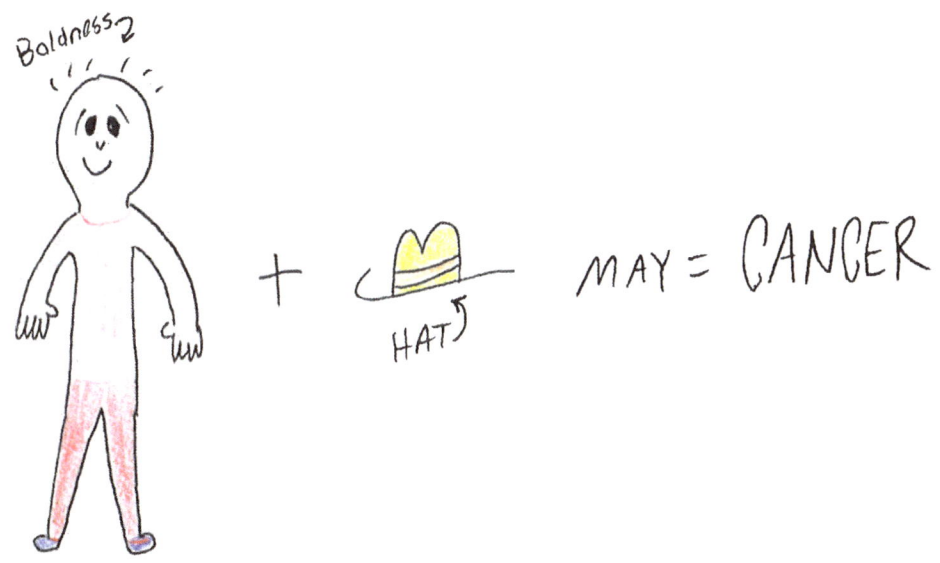

Baldness?

+ HATS MAY = CANCER

After all the treatments and
surgeries are over
        some kids get worried.
They think, "Everyone thinks we're fine now,
            but I am still scared."
You might only see how scary it was
once the hardest part is over.

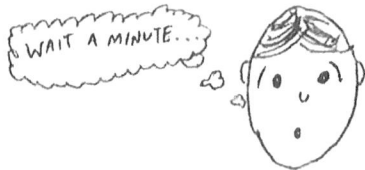

WAIT A MINUTE...

Trust me.
Your mom
    knows.

mom

I CANNOT PROMISE THAT EVERYTHING WILL
BE ALRIGHT. NOR CAN I PROMISE THAT IT WILL
BE OVER FAST AND IT WILL BE AS IF NOTHING
EVER HAPPENED

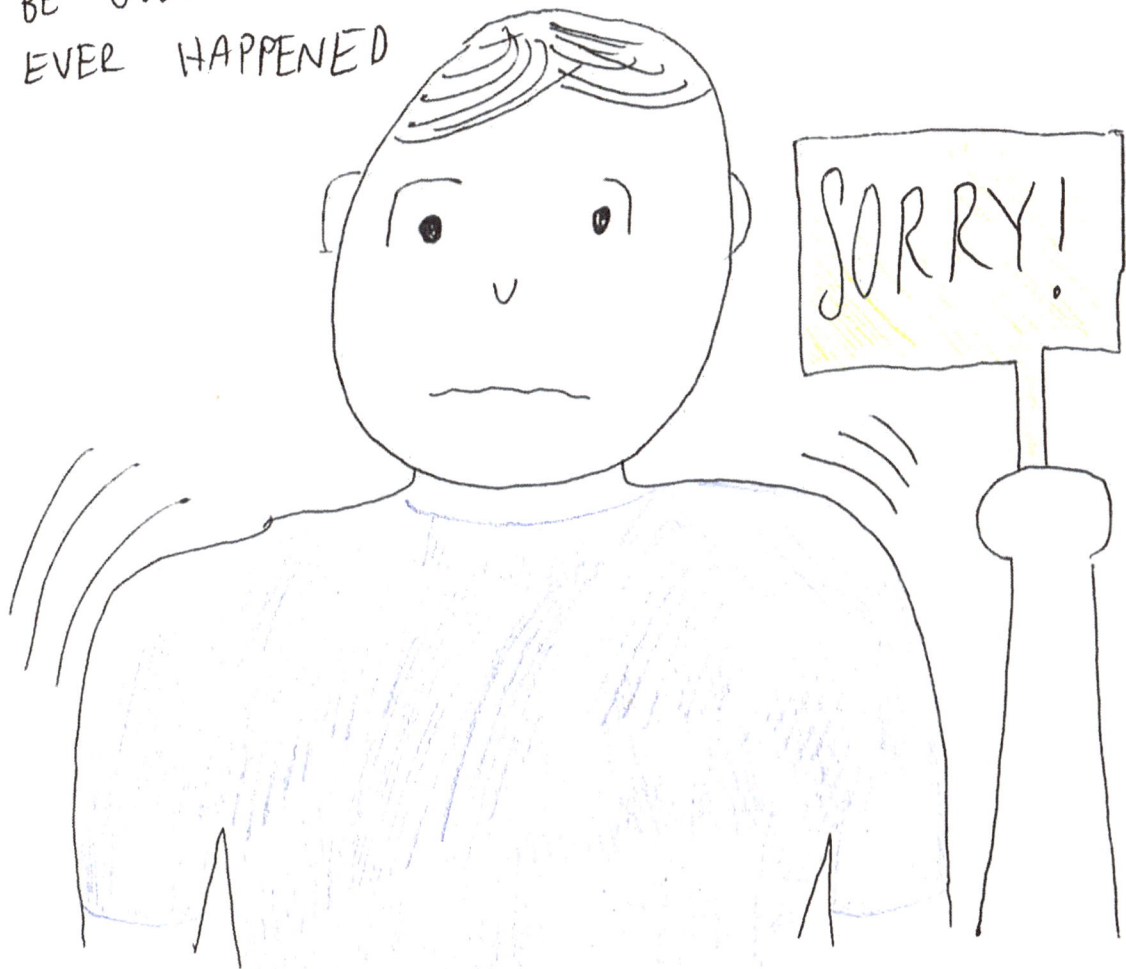

BUT I CAN PROMISE THAT THERE ARE OTHER KIDS GOING THROUGH THE SAME THING THAT YOU ARE GOING THROUGH.

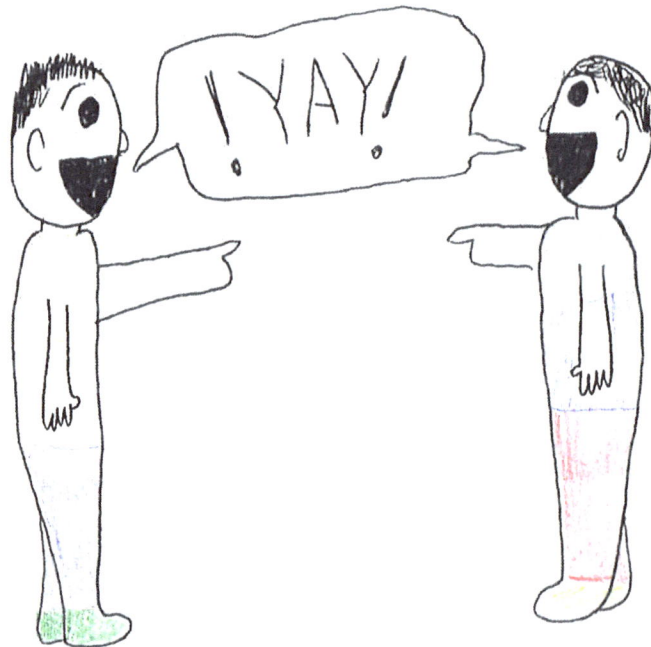

I CAN ALSO PROMISE THAT YOUR PARENT
WILL **LOVE** YOU THROUGHOUT THIS WHOLE
CRAZY JOURNEY.

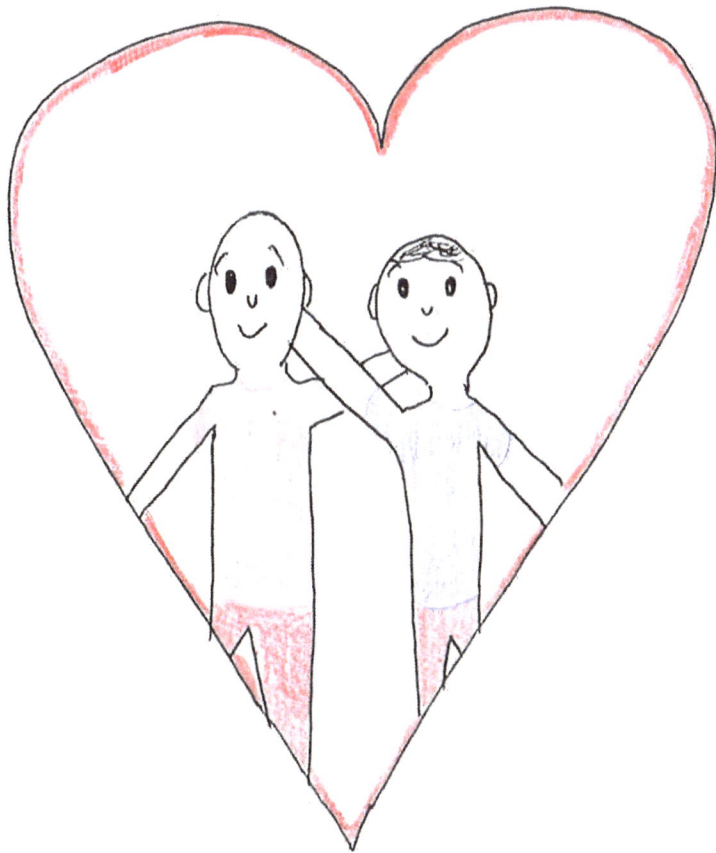

I WISH YOU AND YOUR FAMILY BEST OF LUCK THROUGHOUT THIS EXPERIENCE AND I HOPE THAT EVEN THOUGH THE CANCER JOURNEY CAN BE DIFFICULT AT TIMES, YOU FIND LOVE AND FUN THROUGHOUT IT.

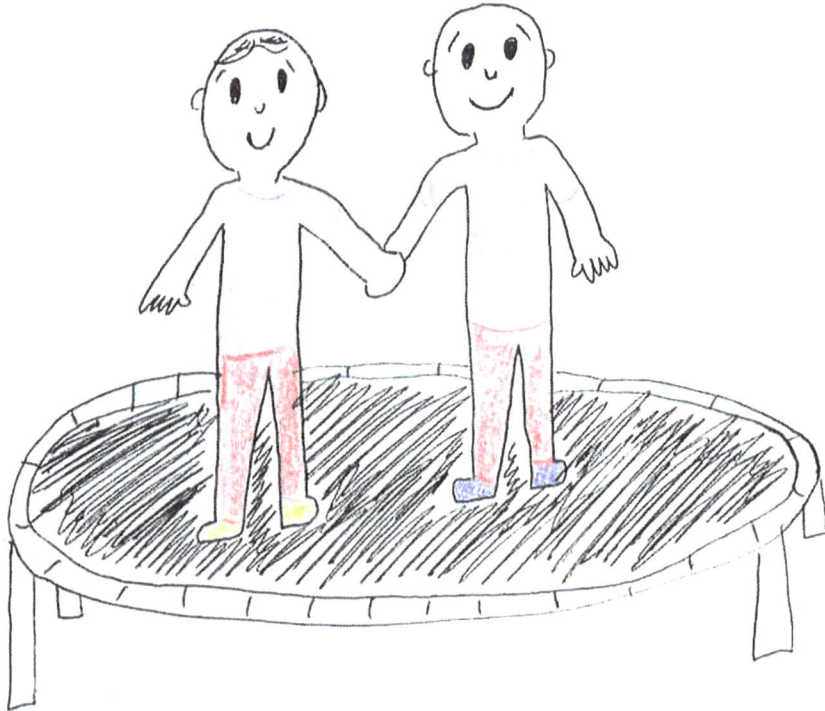

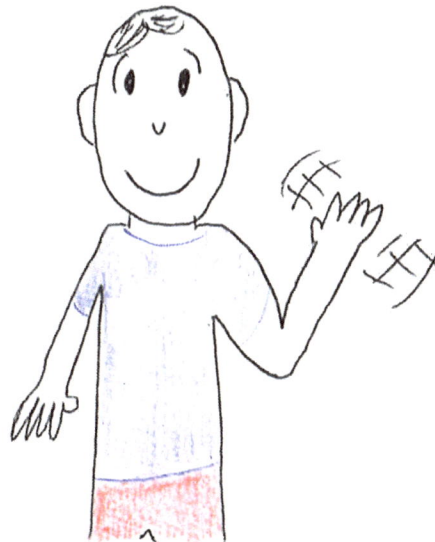

www.ingramcontent.com/pod-product-compliance
Lightning Source LLC
Chambersburg PA
CBHW060806270326

41927CB00002B/72